The Epidemiologist's Apprentice

Your Study Guide on Measures of Disease Occurrence

D. Faulkner Ph.D., MPH

ISBN: 1469912023
ISBN 13: 9781469912028

Dedication

This is dedicated to my departed mentor, MaryFran, who opened my eyes to my gift for teaching and changed the course of my life.

Rest in peace, my dear friend.

Table of Contents

UNIT #1:
Four Mathematical Parameters 1

UNIT #2:
Four Core Epidemiologic Measures 9

UNIT #3:
Five Special Incidence Measures............................ 25

UNIT #4:
Two Equations Linking Measures Together.............. 41

UNIT #5:
One-Year Mortality Rates 49

UNIT #6:
Ratio Measures of Association 61

APPENDIX A:
Graphic Organizers 73

APPENDIX B:
Comprehensive Quiz and Answer Key 79

Preface

Epidemiology is the study of the distribution and determinants of health-related events in human populations, and the application of this study to control health problems. Measures of disease occurrence, such as the prevalence of adult obesity in the United States, are the foundation of this discipline.

This book is a compilation of my lecture outlines and quizzes on the topic of measures of disease occurrence, developed and refined over many years of teaching. These introductory materials may supplement current courses taken by medical and public health students. Public health practitioners may use this book to brush up on their essentials, and my fellow instructors may find this helpful for course development.

Here, I employed instructional design techniques to enhance learning. These techniques include: 1) an emphasis on vocabulary terms; 2) an outline format for easier information processing; 3) self-assessments after each unit, testing declarative and computational knowledge; 4) graphic organizers; and 5) a comprehensive quiz and answer key.

"Practice, the master of all things"
--Augustus Octavius

D. Faulkner

Four Mathematical Parameters

1) **What this unit covers**. This unit introduces four mathematical parameters that provide the building blocks for epidemiologic measures of disease occurrence, the count, ratio, proportion, and rate.

2) **Count**
   a) Definition. The number of cases of a disease or other health phenomena being studied
   b) Notation. n
   c) Examples

      i) The number of cases of influenza reported in Westchester County, New York, during January 2008
      ii) The number of college dorm residents with hepatitis

3) Ratio

a) Definition. One quantity divided by another quantity, whereby there is not necessarily a relationship between the numerator and the denominator

b) Notation. a/b

c) Example

   i) Given one thousand motorcycle fatalities, whereby nine hundred fifty victims are men and fifty are women

   ii) The number of male cases/number of female cases = 950/50 = 19/1

d) Feature. Can be a count divided by a count, a percent divided by a percent, or a rate divided by a rate

4) Proportion

a) Definition. A type of ratio whereby the numerator is included in the denominator

b) Notation. a/(a+b)

c) Feature. Often expressed as a percentage or fraction

d) Example

   i) Given one thousand motorcycle fatalities, whereby nine hundred fifty victims are men and fifty are women

   ii) The proportion of victims who are male = 950/(950 + 50) = 950/1000 = 95 percent

e) Significance

    i) The meaning of a count (numerator) depends on the size of the group it refers to (denominator).

    ii) Say ten college dorm residents have hepatitis (count).

    iii) How large a problem this is depends on the size of the denominator.

    iv) If the dorm houses twenty students, then fifty percent are ill.

    v) If the dorm houses five hundred students, then two percent are ill.

5) Rate

a) Definition. A type of ratio whereby there is a relationship between the numerator and the denominator (like with a proportion), and time is an intrinsic part of the denominator

b) Notation. $a/(a + b)/t$ or $a/[(a + b) \times t]$

    i) Since dividing by something is the same as multiplying by its inverse

    ii) $a/(a + b)/t = [a/(a + b)] \times 1/t$

    iii) $= a/[(a + b) \times t]$

c) Example. Twenty colds per one thousand elementary school students per one-month period

Quiz 1

Instructions: For each numbered item below, specify the **one** most appropriate lettered option. Each lettered option may be selected once, more than once, or not at all.

Questions 1-6.

    a.   Count
    b.   Proportion
    c.   Rate
    d.   Ratio

1. Number of males/number of females

2. Number of males/(number of males + number of females)

3. Weight in kg/height in meters^2 = body mass index

4. Number of children with colds

5. Number of colds/one thousand elementary school students/one-month period

6. Number of fetal deaths/number of conceptions

Instructions: For each numbered item below, specify the **one** most appropriate lettered option.

Questions 7-10.

7. A proportion is a type of ratio.

   a. True
   b. False

8. A rate is a type of ratio.

   a. True
   b. False

9. A count is a type of ratio.

   a. True
   b. False

10. The _____ does **not** necessarily have a numerator and denominator that relate to each other.

    a. Ratio
    b. Proportion
    c. Rate

Quiz 1–Answers

1) d

2) b

3) d

4) a

5) c

6) b

7) a

8) a

9) b

10) a

References

Elandt-Johnson JRC. Definition of rates: some remarks on their use and misuse. Am. J Epidemiol. 1975; 102: 267-271.

Friis RH, Sellers TA. Epidemiology for public health practice. 4th ed. Sudbury: Jones and Bartlett Publishers; 2009.

Granados JAT. On the terminology and dimensions of incidence. J Clin. Epidemiol. 1997; 50: 891-897.

Hennekens CH, Boring JE. Epidemiology in medicine. Boston: Little, Brown and Company; 1987.

Kuzma W, Bohnenblust SE. Basic statistics for the health sciences. 4th ed. New York: McGraw Hill; 2001.

Szklo M, Nieto FJ. Epidemiology beyond the basics. Sudbury: Jones and Bartlett Publishers; 2007.

Four Core Epidemiologic Measures

1) **What this unit covers**. There are two broad categories of epidemiologic measures, prevalence measures and incidence measures. Within these two broad categories are four core measures, the point prevalence, cumulative incidence, incidence density, and period prevalence.

2) **Prevalence**

   a) Definition. Refers to existing disease at a point in time

   b) Significance. Useful for capturing the demand for health services and the burden of disease within a community

3) **Incidence**

   a) Definition. Refers to new disease developing over a period of time

   b) Significance. Useful for exploring cause and effect (called etiologic studies)

4) Point prevalence (P)

a) Definition. The proportion of the population having the disease at a given point in time

b) Feature. Analogous to a single frame of a motion picture or snapshot

c) Calculation. The number of existing cases of disease at a point in time, divided by the total population at that point in time

d) Notation. $P = C(t)/N(t)$

   i) $C(t)$ = count of existing cases at a point in time

   ii) $N(t)$ = total population at a point in time

e) Example

   i) A visual examination survey was conducted in Framingham, Massachusetts, in 2010.

   ii) Among the 2,477 examined, 310 had cataracts.

   iii) The point prevalence is 310/2477, or 12.5 percent.

5) Cumulative incidence (CI)

a) Definition. The proportion of people who become diseased during a specified period of time

b) Features

   i) The "period of time" is called the risk period.

   ii) A synonym for CI is "risk".

c) Calculation. The number of new cases of disease during a time period, divided by the number of disease-free persons at the beginning of the time period

d) Notation. $CI = I(t_0, t) / N(t_0)$

    i) $I(t_0, t)$ = number of new cases from time-zero to time t

    ii) $N(t_0)$ = total disease-free population at time-zero

e) Caveat about the denominator

    i) People must not only be disease-free at time-zero.

    ii) It is implied that people must also be capable of developing the disease.

    iii) For example, in a study of uterine cancer, women with hysterectomies can't be in the denominator.

f) Example

    i) In the Charleston Heart Study, there were 602 males identified as being free of coronary heart disease (CHD).

    ii) During the next fifteen years, 116 people developed CHD.

    iii) The CI of CHD is 116/602 = 19.27 percent over fifteen years.

    iv) Note that the risk period (fifteen years) must be a part of the final answer.

6) Two conditions are required to calculate a CI.

a) There has to be a <u>fixed cohort (or fixed population)</u>, meaning that no new members are allowed to enter the denominator after the start of the study (t_0).

b) There has to be <u>perfect follow-up</u>, meaning that disease status must be determined for everyone in the denominator at the end of the follow-up period (t).

c) Example

   i) At the start of the follow-up period (t_0), you have one hundred disease-free (no hypertension) study subjects.

   ii) At the end of the follow-up period (t) you have the same one hundred study subjects, and each study subject can be classified as hypertensive or non-hypertensive.

7) How might the two conditions be violated, using the example directly above?

a) There is no fixed cohort because new recruits enter the denominator after the study began.

b) There is imperfect follow-up because of <u>attrition</u>, or dropping out, from the denominator.

   i) Possible reasons

      (1) Investigators lose track of study subjects, even though the study subjects did not officially, voluntarily withdraw from the study.

      (2) Study subjects voluntarily withdraw from the study.

   (3) Study subjects die from conditions (e.g., motor vehicle accidents) other than the condition under investigation (hypertension).

  ii) Significance of attrition

   (1) You don't know whether those who are lost would have ultimately ended up in the numerator or not by the end of the follow-up period.

   (2) The longer the follow-up period, the higher the likelihood of attrition.

8) When the two conditions are violated, then what?

 a) You have a <u>dynamic population</u>, a population that is continuously changing, allowing for the addition of new members and the loss of previously entered members.

 b) Instead of counting persons in the denominator, you must count "disease-free time units under observation".

  i) This is called <u>person-time</u> (PT).

  ii) It serves as the denominator of a new measure, called <u>incidence density</u>.

9) Incidence density (ID)

 a) Definition. The average rate of development of disease in a population

b) Example

  i) A hypothetical group of persons was followed for five years (1976-1981).

    (1) Person A was observed from 1/76-1/78, and was then lost to follow-up.

    (2) Person B was observed from 7/76-7/79, and then developed disease.

    (3) Person C was observed from 1/76-1/81, and did not develop disease.

    (4) Person D was observed from 1/77-1/81, and did not develop disease.

    (5) Person E was observed from 1/78-7/80, and then developed disease.

  ii) The total PT is 16.5 person-years (2 years + 3 + 5 + 4 + 2.5).

  iii) The ID = 2 cases/16.5 person-years, or 12.1 cases /100 person-years.

c) Calculation. The number of new cases of disease during a given time period, divided by the summation of each person's time under observation and disease-free

d) Notation. $ID = I(t_0, t)/ \sum \Delta t_i$

  i) $I(t_0, t)$ = number of new cases from time-zero to time t

  ii) $\sum \Delta t_i$ = summation of each person's time under observation and disease-free

e) Feature. There are many types of disease-free time units, such as person-days, person-months, and man-hours.

10) The <u>Big Mac assumption</u> operates with ID.

    a) Definition. Person-time units are equivalent.

        i) For example, 16 person-years can be contributed by 16 persons followed for 1 year, 8 persons observed for 2 years, or 32 persons observed for ½ year; and all of these scenarios are the same.

        ii) This is similar to assuming that eating fifty fast-food hamburgers costing two dollars each is equivalent to eating one one-hundred-dollar filet mignon at the best restaurant in town.

    b) This assumption is reasonable, except with extreme situations (e.g., 100 person-years = 100 persons followed for 1 year = 1 person followed for 100 years).

11) Period prevalence (PP)

    a) Definition. The number of persons who have the disease at any time during the follow-up period, relative to the size of the population for that same period

    b) Feature. Expressed as a percentage

    c) Calculation. The number of prevalent **and** incident cases, divided by the average size of the population

    d) Notation. PP = $(C_o + I)/N^*$

        i) C_o = prevalent cases at time zero

ii) I = incident cases that develop during the time period

iii) N* = average size of the dynamic population during the time period

e) Example

i) A population of one hundred fifty persons was followed for one year, and twenty-five had the disease of interest at the start of the follow-up period.

ii) Another fifteen new cases developed during the year.

iii) The PP = (25+15)/150, or 27 percent.

f) Significance

i) It is employed when it is difficult to determine whether the disease is an existing case or a new case (e.g., mental illness).

ii) It combines prevalence and incidence, so it is **not** used often.

Quiz 2

In a mass screening of 1000 sixty-five-year-old men, 100 were found to have glaucoma. During the following ten-year period, another 200 contracted the disease.

1. What is the prevalence (P) of glaucoma?

    a. 100/900 = 11.1 percent
    b. 100/1000 = 10.0 percent
    c. 200/1000 = 20.0 percent
    d. 200/900 = 22.2 percent

2. What is the ten-year cumulative incidence (CI) of glaucoma?

    a. 100/900 = 11.1 percent
    b. 100/1000 = 10.0 percent
    c. 200/1000 = 20.0 percent
    d. 200/900 = 22.2 percent

In a London area during the years 1970-1973, 832 children were born with a birth weight of <2000g. Of these, 133 were stillborn. Of those born alive, 210 died during the first month after birth.

3. What is the P of being stillborn among those with a birth weight <2000g?

    a. 133/832 = 16 percent
    b. 210/832 = 25 percent
    c. 210/(832-133) = 30 percent
    d. 133/(832-210) = 21 percent

4. What is the CI of death during the first month after birth?

   a. 133/832 = 16 percent
   b. 210/832 = 25 percent
   c. 210/(832-133) = 30 percent
   d. 133/(832-210) = 21 percent

Below are data from a ten-year diabetes incidence study:

Number of subjects (Column A)	Years of observation and disease-free (Column B)	Person-years of observation (Column A x Column B)
20	10	?
10	9	?
7	8	?
2	7	?
1	1	?

5. What is the **total** number of person-years of observation?

   a. 35
   b. 40
   c. 361
   d. 461

6. If the total number of new diabetes cases over a ten-year period is five, what is the incidence density (ID)?

    a. 5/35 = 14.3/100 person-years
    b. 5/40 = 12.5/100 person-years
    c. 5/361 = 1.4/100 person-years
    d. 5/461 = 1.1/100 person-years

In the small study below, on migraines, four patients are followed for a maximum of two years:

Person number	Event	Timing of event	Number of person-years
1	Migraine	At 6 months	?
2	Loss to follow-up	At 1 year	?
3	Migraine	At 1.5 years	?
4	Withdrawal	At 2 years	?

7. What is the total number of person-years of observation?

8. What is the incidence density of migraines?

9. The main difference between point prevalence (P) and cumulative incidence (CI) is that:

    a. P is a proportion, and CI is a rate.
    b. P is a rate, and CI is a proportion.
    c. P requires a fixed cohort, and CI does not.
    d. P refers to a point in time, and CI refers to a period of time.
    e. A and D

10. A difference between cumulative incidence (CI) and incidence density (ID) is that:

    a. CI requires perfect follow-up, and ID does not.
    b. CI is a risk, and ID is a rate.
    c. CI is a rate, and ID is a proportion.
    d. CI refers to a point in time, and ID refers to a period of time.
    e. A and B

11. State the type of population (fixed or dynamic) that best describes each of the following:

    a. People who live in New York City
    b. Men who had coronary bypass surgery as of 2005
    c. Children who were vaccinated against polio in 1955
    d. Women who are practicing physicians

12. At the beginning of 1987, a population size was twenty-four thousand, and at the end of the year, it was twenty-six thousand. At the beginning of 1987, there were ninety-six housebound patients; twenty of these died during 1987, and four moved elsewhere. Another forty people became housebound during 1987, and eight of them died during the year. What is the period prevalence (PP) of being housebound for 1987?

Quiz 2–Answers

1) b

2) d
   200/ (1000-100)

3) a

4) c

5) c

Number of subjects (Column A)	Years of observation and disease-free (Column B)	Person-years of observation (Column A x Column B)
20	10	200
10	9	90
7	8	56
2	7	14
1	1	1
		**Total = 361 person-years

6) c
   5/361 = 0.0138 = 1.38/100 person-years

7) 5

Person number	Event	Timing of event	Number of person-years
1	Migraine	At 6 months	0.5
2	Loss to follow-up	At 1 year	1
3	Migraine	At 1.5 years	1.5
4	Withdrawal	At 2 years	2
		**Total = 5.0 person-years	

8) 2 cases of migraines/5 person-years = 40/100 person-years

9) d

10) e

11) dynamic, fixed, fixed, dynamic

12) $(96 + 40)/[(24,000 + 26,000)/2] = 136/25,000 = 0.0054 = 0.54/100 = 0.54$ percent

References

Abramson JH. Making sense of data: a self-instruction manual on the interpretation of epidemiologic data. New York: Oxford University Press; 1994.

Ahlbom A, Norell S. Introduction to modern epidemiology. Chestnut Hill: Epidemiology Resources Incorporated; 1984.

Aschengrau A, Seage GR. Essentials of epidemiology in public health. Sudbury: Jones and Bartlett Publishers; 2008.

Friis RH, Sellers TA. Epidemiology for public health practice. 4th ed. Sudbury: Jones and Bartlett Publishers; 2009.

Gerstman BB. Epidemiology kept simple: an introduction to traditional and modern epidemiology. Hoboken: Wiley-Liss Incorporated; 2003.

Hennekens CH, Boring JE. Epidemiology in medicine. Boston: Little, Brown and Company; 1987.

Kleinbaum DG, Kupper LL, Morgenstern H. Epidemiologic research: principles and quantitative methods. New York: Van Nostrand Reinhold Company; 1982.

Kleinbaum DG, Sullivan KM, Baker ND. ActivEpi companion textbook: a supplement for use with the ActivEpi CD-ROM. New York: Springer; 2003.

Knapp RG, Miller MC. Clinical epidemiology and biostatistics. Baltimore: Williams & Wilkins; 1992.

Szklo M, Nieto FJ. Epidemiology beyond the basics. Sudbury: Jones and Bartlett Publishers; 2007.

Five Special Incidence Measures

1) **What this unit covers**. There are five special incidence measures, the: a) incidence density census;
   b) one-year incidence rate; c) attack rate; d) case
   fatality rate; and e) survival rate. (See Figure 3-1.)

2) **Introduction to incidence density census**

   a) Recall "incidence density" (ID) from the last unit,
      whereby the denominator is the summation of
      each person's time under observation and dis-
      ease-free; and the numerator is the number of
      new cases over time.

   b) However, summation is not feasible when deal-
      ing with a large, geographically defined popula-
      tion, such as a city.

   c) Therefore, we want to approximate the denomi-
      nator, using the incidence density census.

3) Incidence density census

a) Definition. The average rate of development of disease in a large, geographically defined population

b) Notation. ID census = $I(t_0, t)/(N^* \times t)$

   i) $I(t_0, t)$ = number of new cases from time-zero to time t

   ii) N^* = average size of the dynamic population during the follow-up period, based on census data available close to the chronological time of the study

   iii) t = length of the follow-up period

c) Assumptions

   i) Most persons in the dynamic population are at-risk of disease.

   ii) The dynamic population is in a <u>steady state</u>, meaning that the size and age distribution remain constant over time; there are no major demographic shifts.

d) Example

   i) During a five-year period, two hundred seventy cases of duodenal ulcers occurred in the male population of a city.

   ii) The number of men in the city was eighteen thousand five hundred at the beginning of the period and twenty-one thousand five hundred at the end.

   iii) The ID census = 270/100,000 person-years.

e) Computations for the example directly above

    i) $I = 270$

    ii) $N^* = (18,500 + 21,500)/2 = 20,000$

    iii) $N^* \times t = 20,000$ persons $\times$ 5 years $= 100,000$ person-years

    iv) Therefore ID census $= 270/100,000$ person-years

4) Simplified illustration of how incidence density census can approximate the incidence density (Table 3-1)

a) The disease outcome is death.

b) The initial population size is four.

c) The maximal follow-up period is two years.

d) The ID (of death) $= 2/5$ person-years, or $40/100$ person-years (note that $I = 2$; total person-years $= 5$).

e) The ID census (of death) $= 2/5$ person-years, or $40/100$ person-years (note that $I = 2$; $N^* = [4+1]/2 = 2.5$; $t = 2$ years).

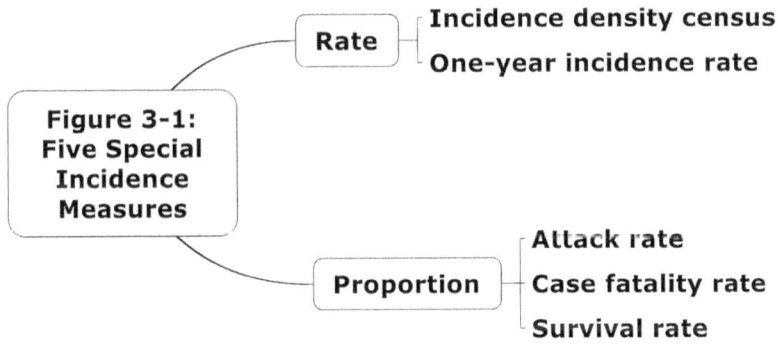

Figure 3-1: Five Special Incidence Measures

Rate
- Incidence density census
- One-year incidence rate

Proportion
- Attack rate
- Case fatality rate
- Survival rate

Table 3-1

Person number	Outcome	Timing of event	Number of person-years
1	Death	At 6 months	0.5
2	Loss to follow-up	At 1 year	1
3	Death	At 18 months	1.5
4	End of study	At 2 years	2.0
			** Total = 5 person-years

5) One-year incidence rate (IR)

a) Definition. The ID census, when the period of observation equals one year

b) Significance. Displayed in government documents

c) Notation. IR = I $(t_0, t)/N^*$

   i) I (t_0, t) = number of new cases from time-zero to time t

   ii) N^* = average size of the dynamic population during the follow-up period (one year), based on census data available close to the chronological time of the study

d) Logic behind the formula directly above

    i) Recall, ID census $= I(t_0, t)/(N^* \times t)$

    ii) If t = one year, the denominator simplifies to N^*

    iii) Now ID census $= I(t_0, t)/N^*$

    iv) The new name is IR

e) Assumptions. Same as those of the incidence density census

f) Example

    i) During a one-year period, two hundred seventy cases of duodenal ulcers occurred in the male population of a city.

    ii) The number of men in the city was eighteen thousand five hundred at the beginning of the period and twenty-one thousand five hundred at the end.

    iii) The IR = 270 cases/20,000 persons, or 14 cases/1,000 persons (note that $I =$ 270; $N^* = [18,500 + 21,500]/2 = 20,000$ persons).

    iv) Also note that there is no person-time in the denominator, as with ID and ID census.

6) Attack rate (AR)

a) Definition. The *cumulative incidence* of disease, observed for limited periods and under special circumstances, as in infectious disease outbreaks

b) Feature. It is **not** a rate like the name says; it is a proportion.

c) Calculation. The number of new cases of disease during a time period, divided by the number of disease-free persons at the beginning of the time period

d) Example

    i) Between 11 pm January 17th and 11 pm January 18th, among a group of one hundred forty medical students attending an end-of-school picnic, ninety contracted food poisoning.

    ii) The AR = 90/140, or 64 percent over the 24-hour period.

7) Case-fatality rate (CFR)

a) Definition. The proportion of individuals with a particular disease who die from that disease, within a specified period of time

b) Feature. It is **not** a rate like the name says; it is a proportion, analogous to the structure of the *cumulative incidence*.

c) Calculation. The number of deaths from a disease, divided by the number of diagnosed patients

d) Example

    i) In 2008, one hundred thirty men living in Florence and Darlington counties suffered myocardial infarctions; sixteen of them died as a result.

    ii) The CFR = 16/130, or 12.3 percent over one year.

8) Survival rate (S)

a) Definition. The proportion of individuals with a particular disease who remain alive from that disease, within a specified period of time

b) Features

    i) It is **not** a rate like the name says; it is a proportion, analogous to the structure of the *cumulative incidence*.

    ii) It is the complement of the CFR.

c) Calculation. 100 percent minus the CFR

d) Example

    i) In 2008, one hundred thirty men living in Florence and Darlington counties suffered myocardial infarctions; sixteen of them died as a result.

    ii) The CFR = 16/130, or 12.3 percent.

    iii) The S = 87.7 percent over one year (100 percent - 12.3 percent).

Quiz 3

1. Which measure does **not** have the "average population" in its denominator?

    a. Incidence density
    b. Incidence density census
    c. Incidence rate

Questions 2-4

A cohort of more than six thousand five hundred elderly people who did not have Parkinson's disease at the start of the study was followed for six years to determine the incidence of new cases of the disease. During the follow-up period, sixty-six participants were diagnosed with Parkinson's disease.

2. The participants contributed 38,458 disease-free person-years. What is the incidence density?

3. How many person-years would have been computed for this study population had not detailed information on each individual's contribution to the total amount of person-years been available?

4. Using the person-years from the previous question, what is the incidence density census?

5. During a four-year period there were 532 new injuries due to accidents among the personnel at certain medical laboratories. The number of

employees was 520 at the beginning of the period and 680 at its end. What is the incidence density census?

6. According to the Swedish Cancer Register, in the years 1991, 1992, and 1993, there were 97, 121, and 112 new cases of pancreatic cancer, respectively, among men between the ages of seventy and seventy-four years. At the beginning of 1991, there were 309,949 men in this age group, and at the end of 1993, there were 332,400 men. What is the incidence density census?

7. In an Asian country with a population of six million people, sixty thousand deaths occurred during the year ending December 31, 1995. These included thirty thousand deaths from cholera among one hundred thousand people who were sick with cholera. What is the case fatality rate (CFR) from cholera in 1995?

Questions 8-9

At the beginning of 1987, a population size was twenty-four thousand; and at the end of the year, it was twenty-six thousand. At the beginning of 1987, there were ninety-six housebound patients; twenty of these died during 1987, and four moved elsewhere. Another forty people became housebound during 1987, and eight of them died during the year.

8. What is the incidence density census of being housebound for 1987?

9. What is the one-year incidence rate of being housebound for 1987?

Questions 10-11

10. In 1998, one hundred thirty individuals living in Westchester County, New York, suffered myocardial infarctions (MI); sixteen of these persons died as a result. What is the 1998 CFR?

11. What is the 1998 survival rate?

Questions 12-16

From the information provided in the table below (food-specific histories of attendees at a luncheon in May 1996), answer the following questions.

	Ate Specific Food			Did Not Eat Specific Food		
Food	Ill	Well	Total	Ill	Well	Total
Ham	11	14	25	26	11	37
Turkey	19	15	34	16	10	26
Potato salad	16	3	19	20	22	42
Pasta salad	10	19	29	17	17	34
Raspberries	33	4	37	4	20	24

12. What is the attack rate (AR) for persons who ate ham?

13. Among persons who ate specific foods, which food had the highest AR?

    a. Ham
    b. Turkey
    c. Potato salad
    d. Pasta salad
    e. Raspberries

14. Overall, which food was eaten least by attendees?

    a. Ham
    b. Turkey
    c. Potato salad
    d. Pasta salad
    e. Raspberries

15. For each food item, if you calculated the cumulative incidence ratio (AR for eaters divided by AR for non-eaters), which food item would have the highest ratio?

    a. Ham
    b. Turkey
    c. Potato salad
    d. Pasta salad
    e. Raspberries

16. Based on your answers to questions 12-15, which food is the most likely source of the food-borne outbreak?

a. Ham
b. Turkey
c. Potato salad
d. Pasta salad
e. Raspberries

Quiz 3–Answers

1) a

2) 66/38,458 = 0.0017 = 17/10,000 person-years; ideally, you want a whole number in the numerator of your final answer

3) 6500 x 6 = 39,000 person-years; this approximates the denominator in question 2 above

4) 66/39,000 person-years = 0.0017 = 17/10,000 person-years

5) 532/{[(520 + 680)/2] x 4} = 532/2400 = 0.22 = 22/100 person-years

6) (97 + 121 + 112)/{[(309,949 + 332,400)/2] x 3} = 330/963,523.5 = 0.00034 = 34/100,000 person-years

7) 30,000/100,000 = 30/100 = 30 percent

8) 40/{[(24,000 + 26,000)/2] x 1 year} = 40/25,000 persons = 0.0016 = 16/10,000 person-years

9) 40/[(24,000 + 26,000)/2] = 40/25,000 persons = 0.0016 = 16/10,000 person-years

10) 16/130 = 0.123 = 12.3 percent

11) 100 percent - 12.3 percent = 87.7 percent

12) 11/25 = 0.44 = 44 percent

13) e

Among eaters: ham = 44 percent; turkey = 56 percent; potato salad = 84 percent; pasta salad = 34 percent; raspberries = 89 percent

14) c

15) e

For each food item, you want to know if eating is a risk factor.

Recall that among eaters, ARs are: ham = 44 percent; turkey = 56 percent; potato salad = 84 percent; pasta salad = 34 percent; raspberries = 89 percent

Among non-eaters, ARs are: ham = 70 percent; turkey = 62 percent; potato salad = 48 percent; pasta salad = 50 percent; raspberries = 17 percent

The largest ratio is raspberries = 89 percent/17 percent = 5.2

16) e

References

Abramson JH. Making sense of data: a self-instruction manual on the interpretation of epidemiologic data. New York: Oxford University Press; 1994.

Ahlbom A, Norell S. Introduction to modern epidemiology. Chestnut Hill: Epidemiology Resources Incorporated; 1984.

Aschengrau A, Seage GR. Essentials of epidemiology in public health. Sudbury: Jones and Bartlett Publishers; 2008.

Gerstman BB. Epidemiology kept simple: an introduction to traditional and modern epidemiology. Hoboken: Wiley-Liss Incorporated; 2003.

Glaser AN. High-yield biostatistics. Philadelphia: Lippincott Williams & Wilkins; 2005.

Gordis L. Epidemiology. Philadelphia: Saunders Elsevier; 2009.

Greenberg RS, Daniels SR, Flanders WD, Eley JW, Boring JR. Medical epidemiology. New York: Lange Medical Books/McGraw-Hill; 2001.

Jekel JF, Katz DL, Elmore JG, Wild SMG. Epidemiology, biostatistics, and preventive medicine. Philadelphia: Saunders Elsevier; 2007.

Kleinbaum DG, Kupper LL, Morgenstern H. Epidemiologic research: principles and quantitative methods. New York: Van Nostrand Reinhold Company; 1982.

Kleinbaum DG, Sullivan KM, Baker ND. ActivEpi companion textbook: a supplement for use with the ActivEpi CD-ROM. New York: Springer; 2003.

Knapp RG, Miller MC. Clinical epidemiology and biostatistics. Baltimore: Williams & Wilkins; 1992.

Last JM. A dictionary of epidemiology. New York: Oxford University Press; 1988.

Szklo M, Nieto FJ. Epidemiology beyond the basics. Sudbury: Jones and Bartlett Publishers; 2007.

Two Equations Linking Measures Together

1) **What this unit covers**. Two mathematical equations describe inter-relationships among previously-discussed measures of disease frequency.

2) **Equation 4-1: P = I x Đ**

   a) P = point prevalence

   b) I = incidence rate (can include incidence density, incidence density census, or one-year incidence rate)

   c) Đ, called "D bar," = <u>average duration of disease</u>

      i) Definition. Average time from disease onset to <u>resolution</u>

      ii) If talking about a fatal disease (e.g., pancreatic cancer), resolution = death

      iii) If talking about a non-fatal disease (e.g., common cold), resolution = recovery

d) Assumption. Steady state

e) Example

    i) From 2003 to 2007, the average annual incidence rate of lung cancer in Connecticut was 45.9 per 100,000, and the average annual prevalence was 23.0 per 100,000.

    ii) What is the average duration of lung cancer?

    iii) The average duration of disease is 0.5 years (Đ = P/I = 23.0/45.9).

3) Why does Equation 4-1 make sense?

a) Say you're sitting in an empty bathtub.

b) When you turn on the faucet and close the drain, the water level rises.

c) The water level drops when you open the drain.

d) Equivalents exist in epidemiology (the <u>epidemiologist's bathtub</u>).

    i) The faucet (or <u>inflow</u>) represents new cases of disease, or incidence.

    ii) The water level represents existing cases of disease, or prevalence.

    iii) The drain (or <u>outflow</u>) represents former cases of disease, or resolution.

    iv) So the message is that prevalence is influenced by inflow and outflow.

4) Why do we care about Equation 4-1?

a) If given two pieces of information, you can solve for the third piece of information. For example, given Ð and incidence data for disease X, you can calculate point prevalence, which you need for health services planning and measuring the burden of disease within a community.

b) It helps you interpret trends.

   i) For example, say you hear on the news that the prevalence of Alzheimer's disease is increasing in the U.S.

   ii) You know that this is not necessarily bad.

   iii) You surmise that inflow has been constant over time, but that newer drugs are keeping patients alive longer (outflow is reduced).

   iv) That is why the prevalence (water level) may be increasing.

5) Equation 4-2: CI = I x t

a) CI = cumulative incidence or risk (proportion)

b) I = incidence rate (can include incidence density, incidence density census, or one-year incidence rate)

c) t = follow-up period length

d) Assumption. Steady state

e) Example

   i) The incidence density of a disease is 5.13/100 person-years.

    ii) What is the estimated cumulative incidence after one year?

    iii) The cumulative incidence is 5.13 percent (5.13 cases/100 person-years x 1 year = 5.13 cases/100 persons).

6) Why does this Equation 4-2 make sense?

a) Given the notation for a rate from Unit 1, $a/[(a + b) \times t]$

b) Multiplying the above by t, yields $a/(a + b)$, which is the notation for a proportion

c) So a rate x t = a proportion

7) Why do we care about Equation 4-2?

a) Often, we want to estimate a risk from a rate.

b) Risks are easier for audiences to understand, particularly lay audiences.

Quiz 4

1. Suppose a treatment is developed that prolongs life but does not result in a cure. How does this affect the incidence of disease?

    a. Incidence increases
    b. Incidence decreases
    c. Incidence is not affected

2. Suppose a treatment is developed that prolongs life but does not result in a cure. How does this affect the prevalence of disease?

    a. Prevalence increases
    b. Prevalence decreases
    c. Prevalence is not affected

3. The prevalence of a disease is decreasing, despite a constant incidence rate. How do you explain this?

    a. The average duration of disease is increasing
    b. The average duration of disease is decreasing
    c. Outflow is increasing
    d. Outflow is decreasing
    e. Both B and C
    f. Both A and D

4. The incidence of a disease over the years has remained stable, at 1/100/year. Its approximate duration (survival after diagnosis) is fifteen years. What is the estimate of the point prevalence?

5. The incidence rate of a nonfatal disease is 500/100,000 person-years. People usually have the disease for an average of three years, at which time the disease resolves spontaneously. Estimate the prevalence of this disease using this information. Assume that the population is in steady state.

Questions 6-7

6. The annual incidence of shingles is 2/100/year, and the average episode of this illness lasts one month. What is the point prevalence?

7. What if a new treatment cuts the duration of an episode of shingles in half but does nothing to prevent shingles from occurring (inflow stays the same)? What is the new prevalence of shingles?

8. The incidence density of a disease is 5.13/100 person-years. What is the estimated cumulative incidence after one year?

Quiz 4–Answers

1) c

2) a

3) e

4) Recall a/(a + b)/t = a/[(a + b) x t]; so 1/100/year = 1/100 person-years; P = I x Đ; P = 1/100 person-years x 15 years = 15/100 persons = 15 percent

5) P = I x Đ; P = 500/100,000 person-years x 3 years = 1500/100,000 persons = 15/1,000 = 1.5 percent

6) P = I x Đ; Đ = 1 month = 1/12 year = 0.083 years; P = 2/100 person-years x 0.083 years = 0.0017 = 0.17/100 persons = 0.17 percent

7) P = I x Đ; Đ = 1/2 month = 1/24 year = 0.042 years; P = 2/100 person-years x 0.042 years = 0.00084 = 0.084/100 persons = 0.084 percent

8) CI = I x t; I x t = 5.13 cases/100 person-years x 1 year = 5.13 cases/100 persons = 5.13%; so when t = 1, cumulative incidence = incidence density

References

Abramson JH. Making sense of data: a self-instruction manual on the interpretation of epidemiologic data. New York: Oxford University Press; 1994.

Ahlbom A, Norell S. Introduction to modern epidemiology. Chestnut Hill: Epidemiology Resources Incorporated; 1984.

Aschengrau A, Seage GR. Essentials of epidemiology in public health. Sudbury: Jones and Bartlett Publishers; 2008.

Gerstman BB. Epidemiology kept simple: an introduction to traditional and modern epidemiology. Hoboken: Wiley-Liss Incorporated; 2003.

Glaser AN. High-yield biostatistics. Philadelphia: Lippincott Williams & Wilkins; 2005.

Jekel JF, Katz DL, Elmore JG, Wild SMG. Epidemiology, biostatistics, and preventive medicine. Philadelphia: Saunders Elsevier; 2007.

Szklo M, Nieto FJ. Epidemiology beyond the basics. Sudbury: Jones and Bartlett Publishers; 2007.

One-Year Mortality Rates

1) **What this unit covers**. This unit explores yet another measure of disease frequency, the one-year mortality rate. There are three broad types: crude, specific, and age-adjusted. The concept of confounding is also introduced.

2) **One-year mortality rate (MR)**

   a) Definition. One-year incidence rate, whereby deaths are measured instead of new disease

   b) Notation. $MR = D(t_0, t)/N^*$

      i) $D(t_0, t)$ = number of deaths from time-zero to time t

      ii) N^* = average size of the dynamic population during the follow-up period (one year), based on census data available close to the chronological time of the study

   c) Assumptions. Same as those for the one-year incidence rate (Unit 3)

d) Significance. Displayed in government documents

e) Feature. Three broad types of one-year mortality rates

    i) <u>Crude</u> (applying to the whole population, without reference to any characteristics of the individuals in it)

    ii) <u>Specific</u> (applying to a subgroup of the population)

    iii) <u>Age-adjusted</u> (crude rates that have been modified to control for the effect of age, to allow for valid comparisons)

3) Crude and specific rates

a) Table 5-1 defines crude and specific rates.

b) Multiplying the numerator and denominator by the <u>multiplier</u> ensures that a whole number ends up in the numerator, for ease of interpretation.

c) The multiplier also helps ensure uniformity across data displays.

d) Example

    i) In 1999, the U.S. had a midyear population of 272,706,000.

    ii) There were 2,391,630 deaths that year.

    iii) The 1999 crude mortality rate is $2,391,630/272,706,000 = 0.00877$.

    iv) Multiply by 100,000 to get a whole integer, 877.

    v) To even things out, divide by 100,000 to get the final answer, which is 877/100,000.

Table 5-1

Name	Numerator	Denominator	Multiplier
Crude mortality rate	Number of deaths during the year	Mid-year population size	1,000 or 100,000
Cause-specific mortality rate	Number of deaths during the year due to a specific cause	Mid-year population size	1,000 or 100,000
Age-specific mortality rate	Number of deaths during the year in a specific age group	Mid-year population size in the same age group	1,000 or 100,000
Race-specific mortality rate	Number of deaths during the year in a specific race group	Mid-year population size in the same race group	1,000 or 100,000
Sex-specific mortality rate	Number of deaths during the year in a specific sex/gender group	Mid-year population size in the same sex/ gender group	1,000 or 100,000

4) Age-adjusted rates (example)

a) You are interested in the effect of climate conditions on mortality.

b) So, you compare the crude mortality rates of Alaska (cold climate) and Arizona (hot climate).

    i) The 2006 crude mortality rate for Alaska was 427/100,000.

    ii) The 2006 crude mortality rate for Arizona was 825/100,000.

c) The conclusion is that Arizona is a more hazardous place to live.

d) But, this conclusion must be questioned, because of the different age distributions of the states (Table 5-2).

    i) Arizona has older residents.

    ii) Older residents are more likely to die than younger residents.

    iii) Therefore, Arizona may have a higher crude mortality rate because the residents are older, not because it has a hot climate.

    iv) Age is a <u>confounder</u>—or distorter—of the climate comparison.

Table 5-2

Age groups	Alaska	Arizona
< 20 years	35 percent	30 percent
20 to 54 years	55 percent	50 percent
55 years and over	10 percent	20 percent

e) The solution is to "erase" the effect of the different age distributions.

    i) Find an age distribution of an external population (e.g., U.S. population in 2000; Table 5-3).

    ii) Mathematically assign Alaska and Arizona the age distribution of the external population.

    iii) Re-compute the Alaska and Arizona mortality rates (computations not shown).

Table 5-3

Age groups	U.S. population in 2000
< 20 years	28 percent
20 to 54 years	52 percent
55 years and over	20 percent

f) Now, you have new <u>age-adjusted</u> mortality rates.

  i) The 2006 age-adjusted mortality rate for Alaska is 856/100,000.

  ii) The 2006 age-adjusted mortality rate for Arizona is 833/100,000.

g) Now, which state is more hazardous?

  i) The answer is Alaska.

  ii) Note that these age-adjusted rates are fictitious, because they depend on the external population used.

  iii) But that is okay because the focus is on comparison not absolute values.

Quiz 5

A total of 2,123,323 deaths were recorded in the U.S. in 1997. The mid-year population was estimated to be 243,401,000. HIV-related mortality and population data by age for all residents and for African-American males are shown below.

1. What is the crude mortality rate?

2. What is the HIV-specific mortality rate for the entire population?

3. What is the HIV-specific mortality rate among thirty-five- to forty-four-year-olds?

4. What is the HIV-specific mortality rate among thirty-five- to forty-four-year-old African-American males?

	All races, all ages		African-American males	
Age group (years)	HIV deaths	Population (x 1000)	HIV deaths	Population (x 1000)
0-34	5756	133,965	1525	9379
35-44	4794	34,305	1212	1663
45-54	1838	23,276	395	1117
>55	1077	51,855	168	1945
Unknown	3		1	
Total	13,468	243,401	3301	14,104

In an Asian country with a population of six million people, sixty thousand deaths occurred during the year ending December 31, 1995. These included thirty thousand deaths from cholera among one hundred thousand people who were sick with cholera.

5. What is the crude mortality rate for 1995?

6. What is the cause-specific mortality rate for cholera in 1995?

The table below presents deaths from coronary heart disease (CHD) among white males participating in the Charleston Heart Study (1988).

7. What is the age-specific mortality rate from CHD for subjects aged fifty-five to sixty-four years?

Age range (y)	Size of population	Deaths from CHD
35-44	243	28
45-54	208	34
55-64	129	39
65-74	55	25
>75	18	7

The table below describes the occurrence of myocardial infarction (MI) among residents of Florence and Darlington counties, South Carolina, 1998.

Population subgroup	Size of population	Number of MI's	Deaths due to MI
White men	17,902	130	16
White women	20,142	35	7
Black men	8,832	17	3
Black women	11,253	11	1
Total	58,129	193	27

8. What is the total cause-specific mortality rate for MI?

9. What is the race- and sex-specific mortality rate for white men?

Quiz 5–Answers

1) 2,123,323/243,401,000 = 0.00872 = 8.72/1,000, or 872/100,000.

2) 13,468/243,401,000 = 5.53 x $10e^{(-5)}$ or 0.0000553 = 5.53/100,000

3) 4794/34,305,000 = 1.40 x $10e^{(-4)}$ or 0.00014 = 14/100,000. This is a cause-specific mortality rate that is also age-specific; that is, the numerator *and* denominator are specific to one age group.

4) 1212/1,663,000 = 7.29x $10e^{(-4)}$ or 0.000729 = 72.9/100,000. This is a cause-specific mortality rate that is also age-, race-, and sex-specific.

5) 60,000/6M = 0.01= 1/100 = 10/1000

6) 30,000/6M = 0.005 = 5/1000

7) 39/129 = 0.302 = 302/1000. This is a cause-specific mortality rate that is also age-specific.

8) 27/58,129 = 0.00046 = 46/100,000. Note that the cause-specific *morbidity* (not necessarily incidence) rate is 193/58,129 = 0.00332 = 332/100,000

9) 16/17,902 = 0.00089 = 89/100,000. This is a cause-specific mortality rate that is also race- and sex-specific.

References

Aschengrau A, Seage GR. Essentials of epidemiology in public health. Sudbury: Jones and Bartlett Publishers; 2008.

Friis RH, Sellers TA. Epidemiology for public health practice. 4th ed. Sudbury: Jones and Bartlett Publishers; 2009.

Gerstman BB. Epidemiology kept simple: an introduction to traditional and modern epidemiology. Hoboken: Wiley-Liss Incorporated; 2003.

Gordis L. Epidemiology. Philadelphia: Saunders Elsevier; 2009.

Jekel JF, Katz DL, Elmore JG, Wild SMG. Epidemiology, biostatistics, and preventive medicine. Philadelphia: Saunders Elsevier; 2007.

Kleinbaum DG, Kupper LL, Morgenstern H. Epidemiologic research: principles and quantitative methods. New York: Van Nostrand Reinhold Company; 1982.

Kleinbaum DG, Sullivan KM, Baker ND. ActivEpi companion textbook: a supplement for use with the ActivEpi CD-ROM. New York: Springer; 2003.

Knapp RG, Miller MC. Clinical epidemiology and biostatistics. Baltimore: Williams & Wilkins; 1992.

Porta M. A dictionary of epidemiology. New York: Oxford University Press; 2008.

U.S. Department of Health and Human Services. Principles of epidemiology in public health practice. 3rd ed. [Internet] Atlanta: Centers for Disease Prevention and Control; [cited 2012 Jan 10]. Available from: http://www.cdc.gov/training/products/ss1000/ss1000-ol.pdf

Ratio Measures of Association

1) **What is unit covers**. Measures of disease frequency (MDF), such as the point prevalence, become even more informative when they are used in a comparative fashion. Here, we explore creating ratios of one measure of disease frequency over another.

2) **The ratio measure of association** (RMA) is defined as the MDF value in the group of interest divided by the MDF value in the comparison group.

   a) Synonyms for the "group of interest" include the "exposed group" and the "index group".

   b) Synonyms for the "comparison group" include the "unexposed group", the "referent group" and the "baseline group".

3) What are the most frequently reported RMA's?

a) The <u>prevalence ratio</u> (PR) is the point prevalence of disease in the exposed group, divided by the point prevalence in the unexposed group.

b) The <u>cumulative incidence ratio</u> (CIR) (or <u>risk ratio</u>) is the cumulative incidence (or risk) of disease in the exposed group, divided by that in the unexposed group.

c) The <u>incidence density ratio</u> (IDR) is the incidence density of disease in the exposed group, divided by that in the unexposed group.

d) The <u>incidence rate ratio</u> (IRR) is the one-year incidence rate of disease in the exposed group, divided by that in the unexposed group.

e) The <u>mortality rate ratio</u> (MRR) is the one-year mortality rate in the exposed group, divided by that in the unexposed group.

4) How are RMA's interpreted?

a) They are interpreted with respect to direction of association, and strength of association.

b) <u>Direction of association</u>. There are three directions of association: positive, negative, and null.

    i) In a <u>positive association</u>, the RMA is greater than 1.0, meaning that the exposed group experiences more of the outcome than the unexposed group. In other words, the exposure is a <u>risk factor</u> for the outcome.

ii) In a <u>negative association</u>, the RMA is less than 1.0, meaning that the exposed group experiences less of the outcome than the unexposed group. In other words, the exposure is a <u>protective factor</u> against the outcome.

iii) In a <u>null association</u>, the RMA equals 1.0, meaning that the exposed group experiences an equal amount of the outcome compared to the unexposed group. In other words, there is no relationship between the exposure and the outcome.

c) <u>Strength of association</u>.

 i) For RMA's greater than 1.0, the higher the ratio value, the stronger the association. The general rule of thumb is as follows (Figure 6-1):

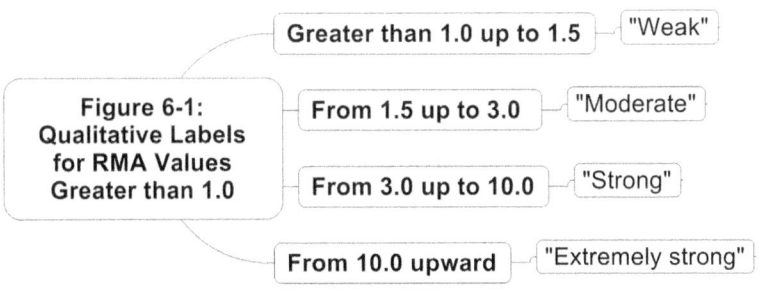

Figure 6-1: Qualitative Labels for RMA Values Greater than 1.0

- Greater than 1.0 up to 1.5 — "Weak"
- From 1.5 up to 3.0 — "Moderate"
- From 3.0 up to 10.0 — "Strong"
- From 10.0 upward — "Extremely strong"

ii) For RMAs less than 1.0, the lower the ratio value, the stronger the association. The scale is as follows (general rule of thumb):

> 0.67 to under 1.0 = Weak
> 0.33 up to 0.67 = Moderate
> 0.10 up to 0.33 = Strong
> Less than 0.10 = Extremely strong

d) Example. In a study of the relationship between smoking and anxiety, 1000 women were classified according to smoking status and current level of anxiety.

  i) The point prevalence of a high anxiety level among smokers is 40%.

  ii) The point prevalence of a high anxiety level among non-smokers is 20%.

  iii) The PR is 40%/20% = 2.

  iv) The direction of association is positive.

   (1) Smokers are 2 times as likely to have a high anxiety level, compared to non-smokers.

   (2) Smoking is a risk factor for a high anxiety level.

  v) The strength of association is moderate.

Quiz 6

Questions 1-12. Late prenatal care is a contributor to poor pregnancy outcomes. In 2005, 16% of White women received late prenatal care, compared with 29% of Black women.

1. What is the Black-White prevalence ratio?

    a. 0.6
    b. 1.8
    c. 0.3

2. In the above ratio, what is the exposed group?

    a. Blacks
    b. Whites

3. In the above ratio, what is the unexposed group?

    a. Blacks
    b. Whites

4. In the above ratio, what is the direction of association?

    a. Positive
    b. Negative
    c. Null

5. In the above ratio, what is the strength of association?

    a. Strong
    b. Moderate
    c. Weak

6. If the above ratio were 1.8, how would it be interpreted?

   a. The point prevalence of late prenatal care among Black women is 1.8 times the point prevalence of late prenatal care among White women.

   b. The point prevalence of late prenatal care among White women is 1.8 times the point prevalence of late prenatal care among Black women.

   c. Black race is a risk factor for late prenatal care.

   d. White race is a risk factor for late prenatal care.

   e. A and C

   f. B and D

7. What is the White-Black prevalence ratio?

   a. 0.6
   b. 1.8
   c. 0.3

8. In the above ratio (Question #7), what is the exposed group?

   a. Blacks
   b. Whites

9. In the above ratio (Question #7), what is the unexposed group?

   a. Blacks
   b. Whites

10. In the above ratio (Question #7), what is the direction of association?

    a. Positive
    b. Negative
    c. Null

11. In the above ratio (Question #7), what is the strength of association?

    a. Strong
    b. Moderate
    c. Weak

12. If the above ratio (Question #7) were 0.3, how would it be interpreted?

    a. The point prevalence of late prenatal care among Black women is 0.3 times (3/10) the point prevalence of late prenatal care among White women.

    b. The point prevalence of late prenatal care among White women is 0.3 times (3/10) the point prevalence of late prenatal care among Black women.

    c. White race is a protective factor against late prenatal care.

    d. Black race is a protective factor against late prenatal care.

    e. A and D

    f. B and C

Questions 13-14.

Pellagra is a disease caused by dietary deficiency of niacin and characterized by dermatitis, diarrhea, and dementia. The 10-year risk of this disease among mill workers was 0.9%. The risk of disease among those who did not work in the mill was 4.4%.

13. What is the risk ratio of pellagra for mill workers versus non-mill workers?

    a. 4.9
    b. 0.2
    c. 3.5

14. If the risk ratio directly above were 0.2, how would it be interpreted?

    a. The risk of pellagra among mill workers is 0.2 times (1/5) the risk of pellagra among non-mill workers.

    b. The risk of pellagra among non-mill workers is 0.2 times (1/5) the risk of pellagra among mill workers.

    c. Non-mill working is a protective factor against pellagra.

    d. Mill working is a protective factor against pellagra.

    e. A and D

    f. B and C

15. The 10-year risk of developing epilepsy among smokers was 5%. The same risk among non-smokers was 5%. What is the direction of association?

a. Positive
b. Negative
c. Null

Quiz 6–Answers

1) b

   0.29/0.16 = 1.81

2) a

3) b

4) a

5) b

6) e

7) a

   0.16/0.29 = 0.55

8) b

9) a

10) b

11) b

12) f

13) b

   0.009/0.044 = 0.2

14) e

15) c

References

Gerstman BB. Epidemiology kept simple: an introduction to traditional and modern epidemiology. Hoboken: Wiley-Liss Incorporated; 2003.

Knapp RG, Miller MC. Clinical epidemiology and biostatistics. Baltimore: Williams & Wilkins; 1992.

U.S. Department of Health and Human Services. Principles of epidemiology in public health practice. 3rd ed. [Internet] Atlanta: Centers for Disease Prevention and Control; [cited 2012 Jan 10]. Available from: http://www.cdc.gov/training/products/ss1000/ss1000-ol.pdf

Appendix A:
Graphic Organizers

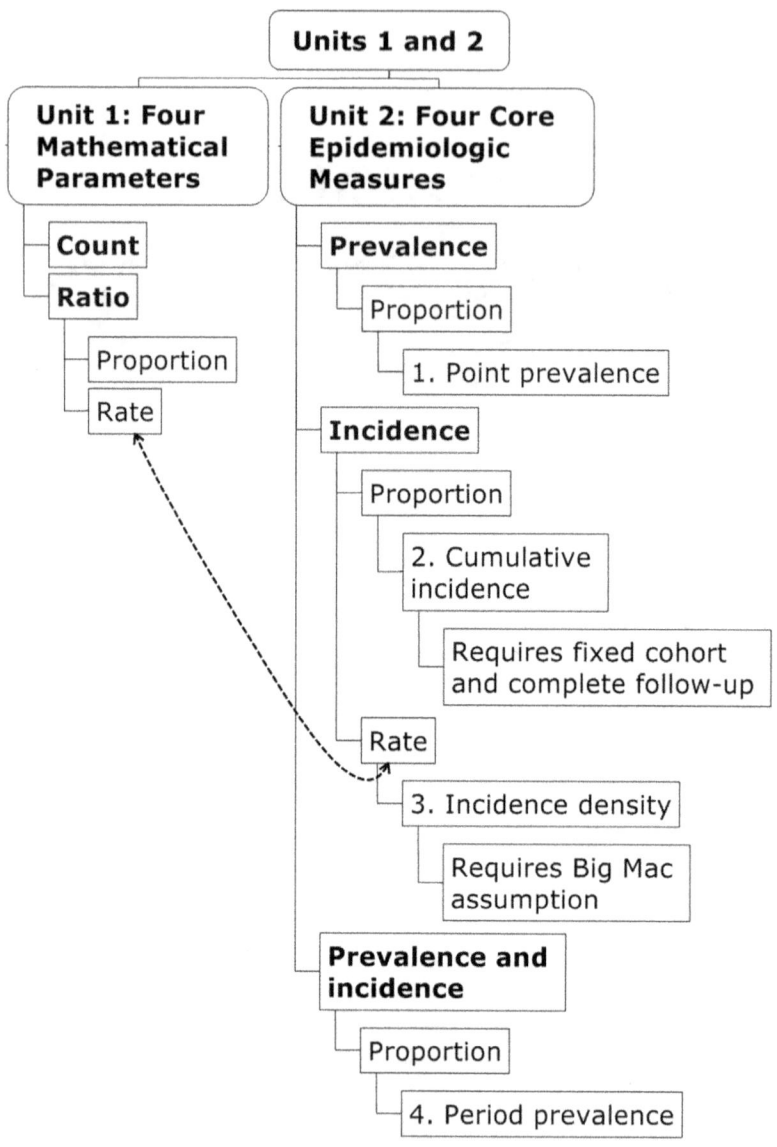

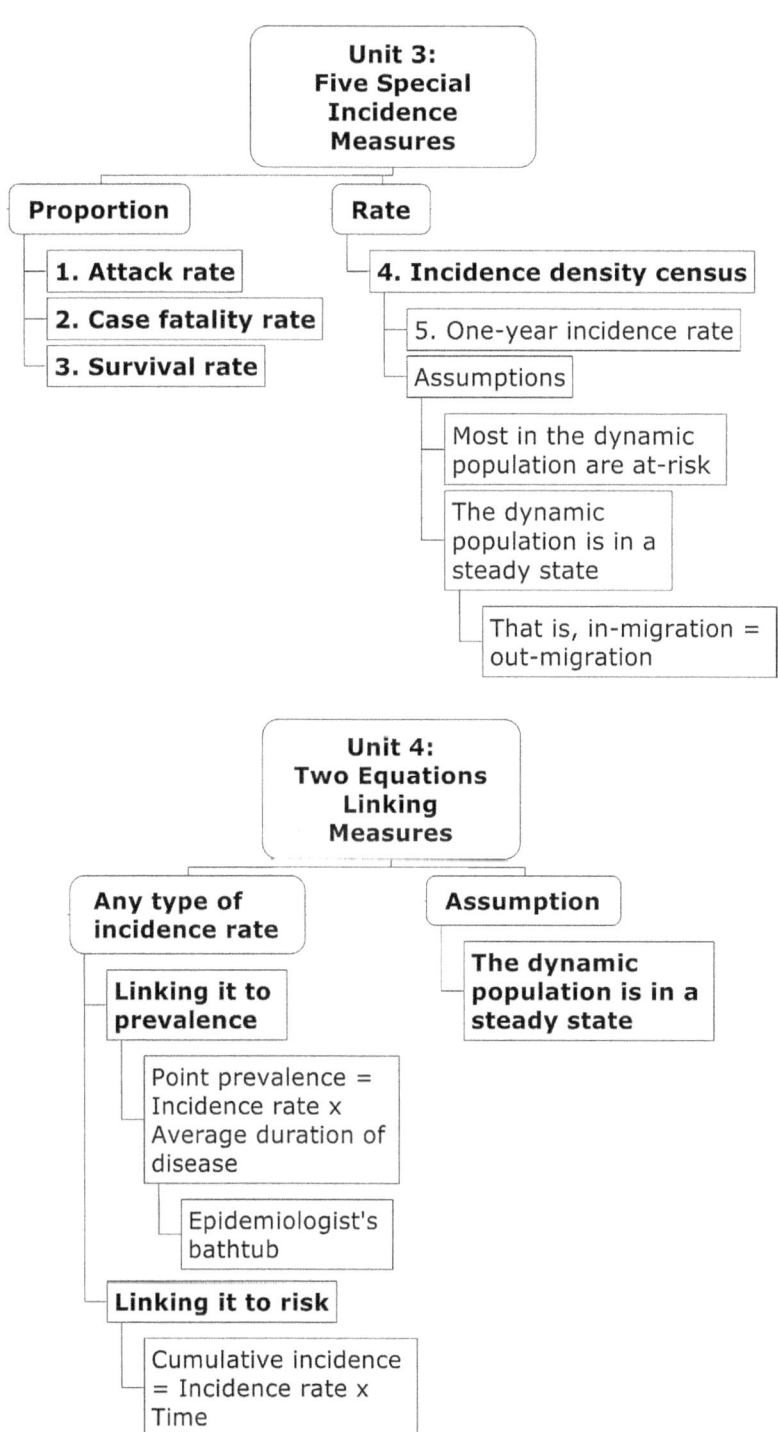

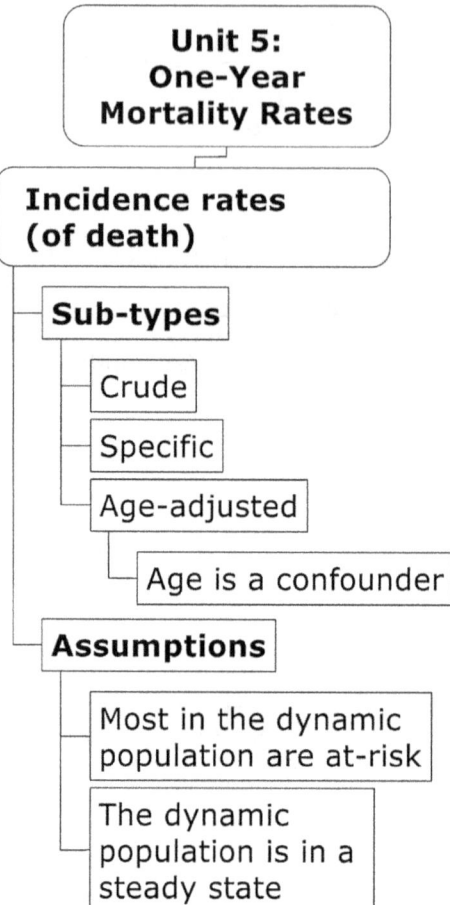

**Unit 5:
One-Year
Mortality Rates**

**Incidence rates
(of death)**

Sub-types

Crude

Specific

Age-adjusted

Age is a confounder

Assumptions

Most in the dynamic
population are at-risk

The dynamic
population is in a
steady state

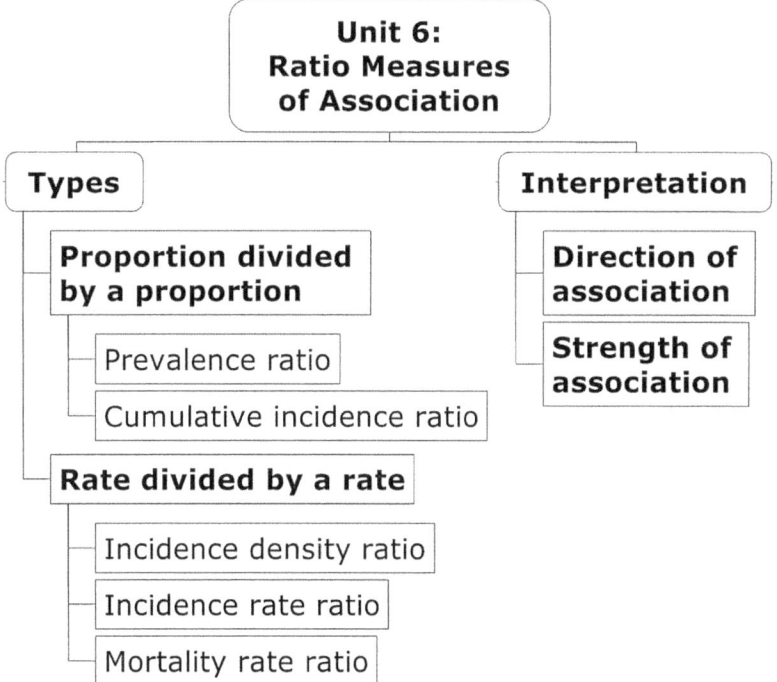

Appendix B:
Comprehensive Quiz
and Answer Key

Comprehensive Quiz

Instructions: For each numbered item below, specify the **one** most appropriate lettered option. Each lettered option may be selected once, more than once, or not at all.

Questions 1-4

a.   This is a use primarily for incidence data.
b.   This is a use primarily for prevalence data.
c.   This application could apply equally for both incidence and prevalence data.
d.   This is a use for neither incidence nor prevalence data.

1.   For determining workload and planning the scope of facilities and manpower needs, particularly in chronic disease

2.   The fundamental tool for etiologic studies of both acute and chronic diseases

3.   To express the burden or extent of some condition or attribute in a population

4.   To provide a direct estimate of the risk of developing a disease

Questions 5-12

a.   Proportion
b.   Rate

5. Point prevalence

6. Cumulative incidence

7. Period prevalence

8. Incidence density census

9. Attack rate

10. Case fatality rate

11. Survival rate

12. Crude death rate

Questions 13-17

a. True
b. False

13. In a fixed cohort, you gain no new members, although you may lose some existing members to death.

14. Given a dynamic population, it is better to calculate a risk than an incidence density.

15. The Big Mac assumption is a reasonable assumption most of the time.

16. When the duration of a disease becomes short and the incidence is high, the prevalence becomes similar to incidence.

17. For a chronic disease of low incidence and long duration, prevalence of the disease increases relative to incidence.

Instructions: For each numbered item below, specify the **one** most appropriate lettered option.

Questions 18-21

Santa Elena is a seacoast community with a population of ninety-nine thousand. Its residents can be divided into three age ranges: twenty-five to forty-four, forty-five to sixty-four, and sixty-five and older—each comprising one-third of the population. In 1990, one hundred cases of hepatitis A occurred in Santa Elena and were traced to the consumption of contaminated oysters. Of these one hundred cases, twenty between the ages of twenty-five and forty-four, ten between the ages of forty-five and sixty-four, and five over the age of sixty-four ultimately proved fatal. Prior to 1990, Santa Elena had never reported a case of hepatitis A.

18. What is the 1990 crude mortality rate for hepatitis A in Santa Elena?

a. 350 per 1000
b. 1.01 per 1000
c. 3.54 per 10,000
d. 1.06 per 1000
e. Cannot be determined from the data

19. What was the incidence of hepatitis A in 1990 (assuming no cases of the disease occurred in Santa Elena prior to 1990)?

    a. 0.00101
    b. 0.00035
    c. 0.35
    d. 0.04
    e. Cannot be determined from the data

20. What is the age-specific mortality rate for residents over sixty-four years of age?

    a. 3.03 per 10,000
    b. 4.55 per 10,000
    c. 6.06 per 10,000
    d. 3.54 per 10,000
    e. 1.52 per 10,000

21. What is the case fatality rate for hepatitis A in Santa Elena?

    a. 3.03 per 10,000
    b. 3.54 per 10,000
    c. 350 per 1000
    d. 1.01 per 1000
    e. Cannot be determined from the data

Comprehensive Quiz–Answers

1) b

2) a

3) b

4) a

5) a

6) a

7) a

8) b

9) a

10) a

11) a

12) b

13) a

14) b

15) a

16) a

17) a

18) c

$$(20 + 10 + 5)/99{,}000 = 0.000354 = 3.54/10{,}000$$

19) a

100/(99,000 x 1) = 0.00101

20) e

5/33,000 = 0.000152 = 1.52/10,000

21) c

(20+10+5)/100 = 35/100 = 350/1000

References

Friis RH, Sellers TA. Epidemiology for public health practice. 4th ed. Sudbury: Jones and Bartlett Publishers; 2009.

Knapp RG, Miller MC. Clinical epidemiology and biostatistics. Baltimore: Williams & Wilkins; 1992.

About the Author

Dr. Faulkner is a professor who resides in Pennsylvania. Both of her graduate degrees are in epidemiologic science.

www.ingramcontent.com/pod-product-compliance
Lightning Source LLC
Chambersburg PA
CBHW051344170526
45166CB00002B/946